Countering Early Aging and Promoting General Wellbeing: A Holistic Guide To Living Youthfully

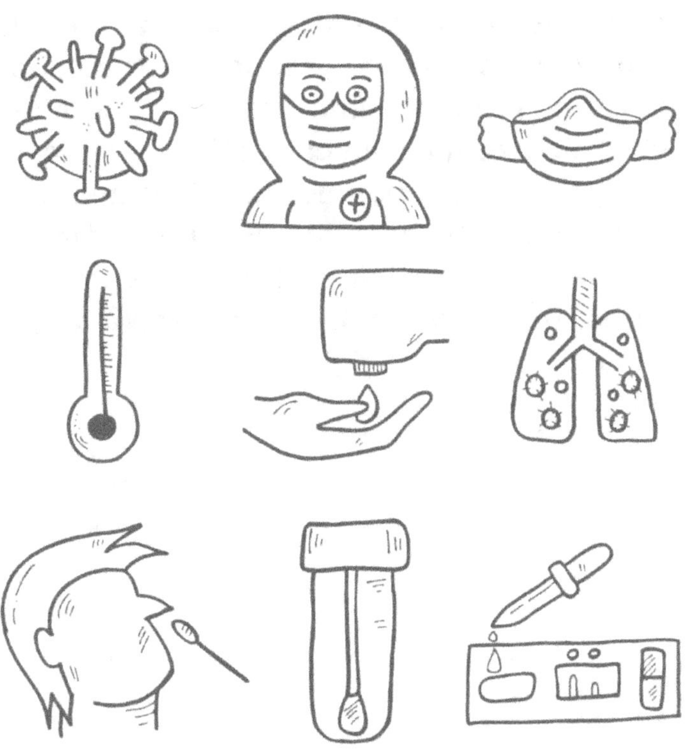

By
BROWN STEVE

INTRODUCTION

Introduction to Countering Early Aging and Promoting General Wellbeing. In our fast-paced society, many individuals are seeking ways to counter early ageing and enhance their overall wellbeing. The desire to live a vibrant and fulfilling life has led to increased interest in effective strategies that promote longevity and vitality. This introduction aims to provide an overview of the importance of general wellbeing in countering early ageing and how adopting a holistic approach can contribute to a healthier and more youthful life.

Early aging can manifest in various forms, including physical, mental, and emotional decline. Factors such as stress, poor nutrition, sedentary lifestyles, and environmental pollutants can accelerate the aging process. However, by prioritizing general wellbeing, individuals can proactively address these factors and mitigate their impact.

General wellbeing encompasses multiple dimensions, including physical, mental, emotional, social, and spiritual aspects of life. It is an integrative approach that recognizes the interdependence of these dimensions and the need for balance and harmony. By considering and nurturing each dimension, individuals can pave the way towards a more vibrant and resilient existence.

Maintaining physical health is a crucial pillar of general wellbeing. Regular exercise, proper nutrition, sufficient sleep, and adequate hydration are essential factors in countering early aging. Engaging in cardiovascular exercises, strength training, and flexibility routines can help maintain muscle tone, bone density, and cardiovascular health.

A balanced and nutrient-dense diet rich in antioxidants, vitamins, and minerals can provide the necessary fuel for cell rejuvenation and support various body functions. Sufficient restorative sleep allows the body to repair and regenerate, while hydrating adequately ensures optimal cellular function and healthy skin.

Caring for mental and emotional health is equally vital in promoting general wellbeing and countering early aging. Chronic stress, anxiety, and negative emotions can accelerate aging processes. Practices such as mindfulness, meditation, and stress management techniques can help reduce stress levels, improve cognitive function, and enhance emotional resilience. Cultivating positive self-talk, engaging in activities that bring joy and fulfillment, and seeking support from friends, family, or professionals can contribute to a healthier mental and emotional state.

Social connections play a pivotal role in general wellbeing and combating early aging. Building and nurturing meaningful relationships promotes feelings of belonging, support, and connectedness, which are fundamental to overall happiness and emotional wellbeing. Engaging in social activities, participating in group hobbies, and joining communities that align with personal interests can provide a sense of purpose and satisfaction that contributes to a youthful and fulfilling life.

Furthermore, nurturing spiritual wellbeing can bring profound benefits to countering early aging. Exploring and finding meaning in life, connecting with something larger than oneself, practicing gratitude and compassion, and expressing personal values and beliefs can provide inner peace and a sense of purpose. Cultivating a spiritual practice, whether through meditation, prayer, or engaging with nature, can enhance overall wellbeing and promote a vibrant and youthful state of being.

Lastly, countering early aging and promoting general wellbeing require a holistic approach that encompasses physical, mental, emotional, social, and spiritual dimensions of life. By prioritizing each aspect and adopting lifestyle habits that support overall health, individuals can optimize their wellbeing and enjoy the benefits of a more vibrant and youthful existence. Embracing this comprehensive approach can empower individuals to take control of their aging process and lead a life filled with vitality, joy, and fulfilment.

CHAPTER ONE

The Biology of Senescence in Aging

Entropy is the ultimate winner
There is a limited amount of time that each multicellular creature may develop and preserve its identity utilizing solar energy. The organism then ages as degradation takes precedence over production. The time-related decline of physiological processes required for reproduction and survival is known as aging. All members of a species are impacted by the traits of aging, as opposed to aging-related disorders like cancer and heart disease.

Maximum Life Span and Life expectation
The maximum life span is a specific of the species. It's the maximum number of times a member of that species has been known to survive. The maximum mortal life span is estimated to be 121 times. The life spans of tortoises and lake trout are both unknown, but are estimated to be further than 150 times. The maximum life span of a domestic canine is about 20 times, and that of a laboratory mouse is 4.5 years.

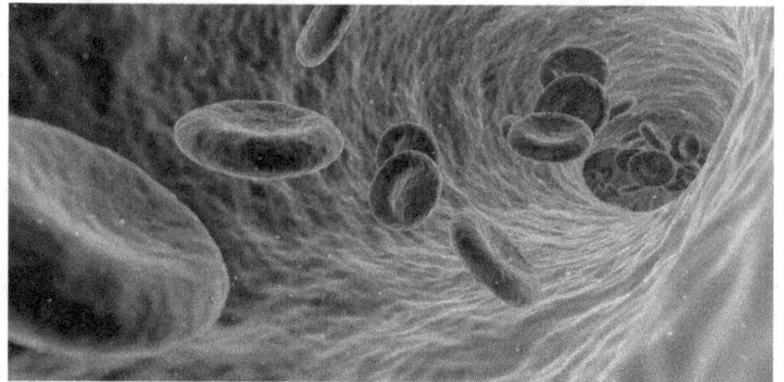

However, over 90 bones as naiads, it has a maximum life span of 3 months, If a Drosophila fruit cover survives to eclose(in the wild. still, a person can not anticipate to live 121 times, and utmost mice in the wild don't live to celebrate their first birthday.

The life expectation, the quantum of time a member of a species can anticipate to live, isn't characteristic of species, but of populations. It's generally defined as the age at which half the population still survives. A baby born in England in the 1780s could anticipate to live to be 35 times old. In Massachusetts during that same time, the life expectation was 28 times.

This was the normal range of mortal life expectancy for the utmost of the mortal race in utmost times. Indeed, the life expectancy in some areas of the world(Cambodia, Togo, Afghanistan, and several other countries) is lower than 40 times. In the United States, a child born in 1986 can anticipate to live 71 times if manly and 78 times if womanish.

Given that in utmost times and places, humans didn't live important past 40 times, our mindfulness of mortal aging is fairly new. A 65-time-old person was rare in social America, but is a common sight moment.. In 1900, 50% of American women were dead by age 58. In 1980, 50% of American women were dead by age 81. therefore, the marvels of anility and the conditions of aging are much more common moment than they were a century agone.

In 1900, people didn't have the " luxury " of dying from heart attacks or cancers. These conditions generally do in people over the age of 50. Rather, people failed(as they're still dying in numerous corridors of the world) from contagious conditions and spongers.

Also, until lately, fairly many people displayed the more general mortal sensecent phenotype graying hair, sagging and wrinkling skin, common stiffness, osteoporosis(loss of bone calcium), loss of muscle filaments and muscular strength, memory loss, sight deterioration and the slowing of sexual responsiveness. As Shakespeare noted in As You Like It, those who did survive to anility left the world " sans teeth, sans eyes, sans taste, sans everything

CHAPTER TWO

Causes of Aging

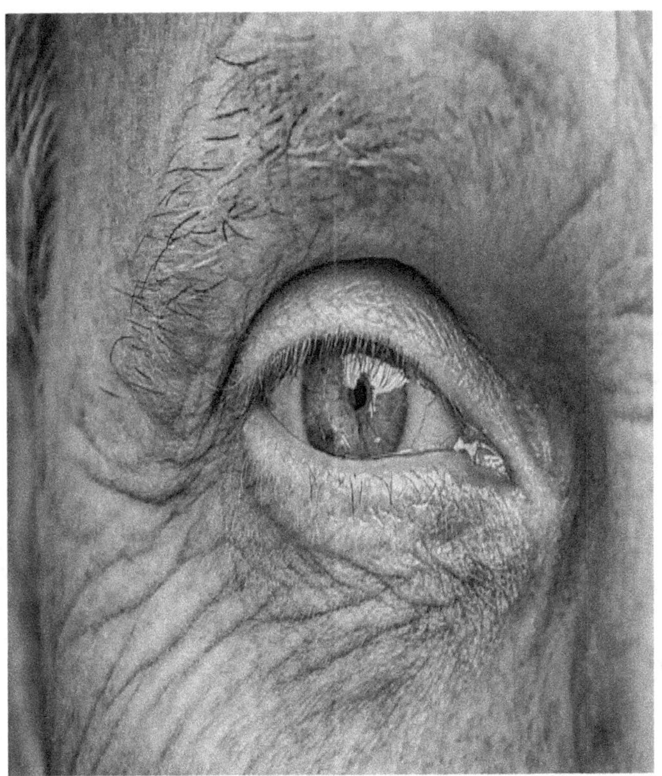

The general ancient phenotype is characteristic of each species. But what causes it? This question can be asked at numerous situations. We'll be looking primarily at the cellular position of association. Indeed then, there's substantiation for numerous different propositions, and there isn't yet a agreement on what causes aging. Oxidative damage One major proposition sees our metabolism as the cause of our aging.

According to this proposition, aging is a by-product of normal metabolism; no mutations are needed. About 2 – 3 of the oxygen tittles taken up by the mitochondria are reduced rightly to reactive oxygen species (ROS). These ROS include the superoxide ion, the hydroxyl revolutionary, and hydrogen peroxide. ROS can oxidize and damage cell membranes, proteins, and nucleic acids. substantiation for this proposition includes the observation that Drosophila that overexpress enzymes that destroy ROS(catalase, which degrades peroxide, and superoxide dismutase) live 30 – 40 longer than do controls.

Also, flies with mutations in the methuselah gene(named after the Biblical fellow said to have lived 969 times) live 35 longer than wild-type canvases . The methuselah mutants have enhanced resistance to paraquat, a bane that works by generating ROS within cells. These findings not only suggest that aging is under inheritable control, but also give substantiation for the part of ROS in the aging

process. The substantiation for ROS
involvement in mammalian aging isn't as clear.

Mutations in mice that affect in the lack of
certain ROS- demeaning enzymes don't beget
unseasonable aging. Still, there may be more
inheritable redundancy in mammals than in
pets, and other genes may be over- regulated
to produce related ROS- demeaning enzymes.
Migliaccio and associates(1999) have
observed mutant mice that live one- third
longer than their wild- type littermates. These
mice warrant a particular protein, p66shc. They
develop typically, but the lack of p66shc
supposedly gives them cellular resistance to
ROS, and therefore advanced resistance to
oxygen- convinced stress on membranes and
proteins.

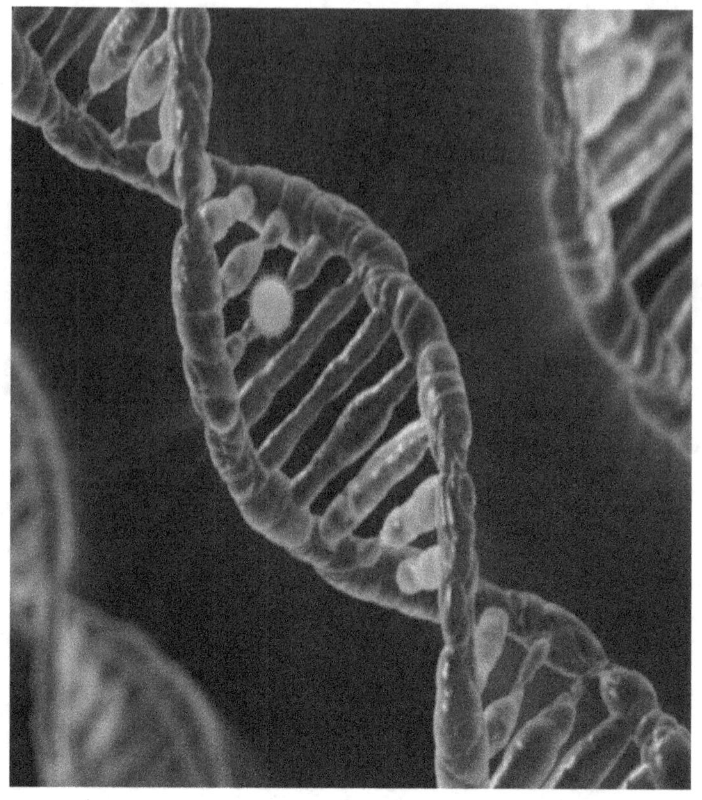

The p66shc protein may be a element of a signal transduction pathway that leads to apoptosis upon oxygen stress, and it may be involved in interceding the life spans of mammals.

Another type of substantiation does suggest that ROS may be important in mammalian aging growing in mammals can be braked by sweet restriction.. Still, sweet restriction can also have other goods, so it isn't certain if it works by precluding ROS conflation. Also, vitamins E and C are both ROS impediments, and vitamin E increases the life of canvases and nematodes when it's added to their diet. Still, results in mammals aren't as easy to interpret, and there's no clear substantiation that ROS impediments work as well as in pets. General wear- and- gash and inheritable insecurity " Wear- and- gash " propositions of aging are among the oldest suppositions proposed to regard the general scenescent phenotype.

As one gets aged, small traumas to the body make up. Point mutations increase in number, and the edge of the enzymes decoded by our genes drop. also, if a mutation occurs in a part of the protein synthetic outfit, the cell would have a large chance of defective proteins.

Still, the rate of mutations would be anticipated to increase markedly, have proved similar defective DNA polymerases in ancient cells, If mutations arose in the DNA- synthesizing enzymes. Likewise, DNA form may be important in precluding anility, and species whose members' cells have more effective DNA form enzymes live longer.

CHAPTER THREE

Mitochondrial genome damage

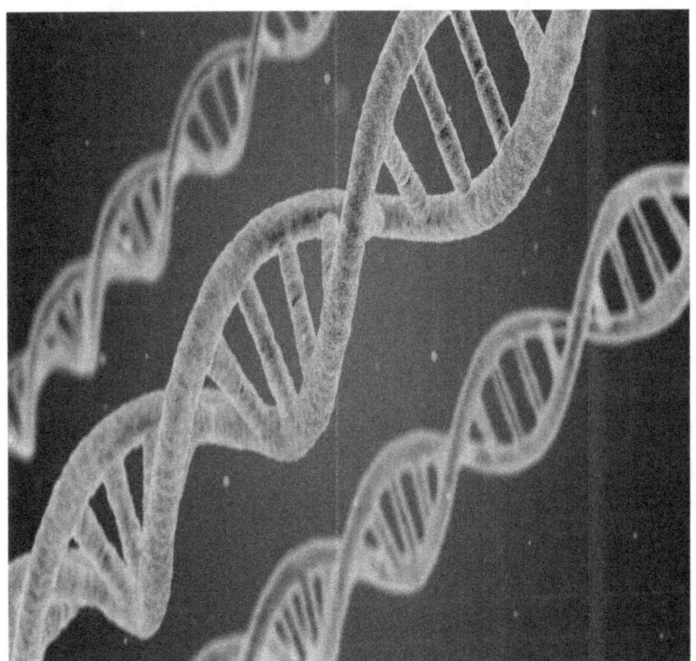

The mutation rate in mitochondria is 10 – 20 times faster than the nuclear DNA mutation rate. It's allowed that mutations in mitochondria could
(1) lead to scars in energy product,
(2) lead to the product of ROS by imperfect electron transport,
(3) induce apoptosis.

Age-dependent declines in mitochondrial function are seen in multitudinous brutes, including humans. A recent report shows that there are " hot spots " for age- related mutations in the mitochondrial genome, and that mitochondria with these mutations have a more advanced replication frequency than wild- type mitochondria. Thus, the mutants are suitable to outcompete the wild- type mitochondria and eventually dominate the cell and its progeny. Also, the mutations may not only allow farther ROS to be made, but may make the mitochondrial DNA more susceptible to ROS- interceded damage.

CHAPTER FOUR

Telomere shortening

Telomeres are repeated DNA sequences at the ends of chromosomes. They are not replicated by DNA polymerase, and they will dock at each cell division unless maintained by telomerase. Telomerase adds the telomere onto the chromosome at each cell division.

The utmost mammalian physical apkins warrant telomerase, so it has been proposed(Salk 1982; Harley et al. 1990) that telomere shortening could be a " timer " that eventually prohibits the cells from dividing any farther. When mortal fibroblasts are dressed, they can divide only a certain number of times, and their telomeres shorten.

However, they can continue dividing(Bodnar et al, If these cells are made to express telomerase. 1998; Vaziri and Benchimol 1998). still, there is no correlation between telomere length and the life span of an beast(humans have shorter telomeres than mice), nor is there a correlation between mortal telomere length and a person's age (Cristofalo et al. 1998).

Telomerase-deficient mice do not show profound aging scars, which we would anticipate if telomerase were the major factor in determining the rate of aging(Rudolph etal. 1999). It has been suggested that telomere-dependent inhibition of cell division might serve primarily as a defense against cancer rather than as a kind of " growing timer. " heritable aging programs Several genes have been shown to affect aging.

In humans, Hutchinson- Gilford progeria pattern causes children to progress swiftly and to die(generally of heart failure) as early as 12 times. It's caused by a dominant mutant gene, and its symptoms include thin skin with age spots, resorbed bone mass, hair loss, and arteriosclerosis. A similar pattern is caused by mutations of the klotho gene in mice(Kuro- o et al. 1997). The functions of the products of these genes are not known, but they are allowed to be involved in suppressing the aging phenotypes. These proteins may be extremely important in determining the timing of juvenility.

CHAPTER FIVE

Achieving overall Heartiness requires a comprehensive approach that focuses on colorful aspects of life. Then is an expansive approach to heartiness.

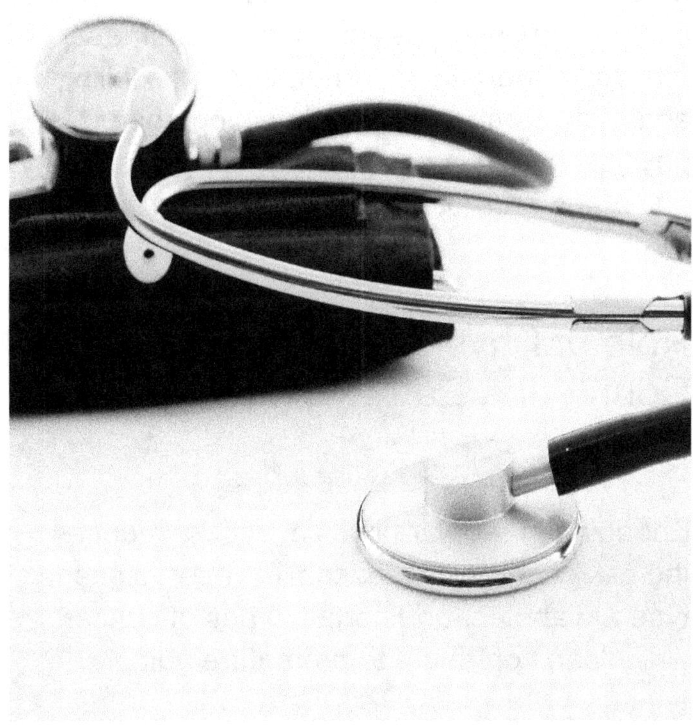

PHYSICAL HEALTH

Explanation of Physical Health

Physical health simply mean the overall well-being of an individual's body and its ability to function optimally. It encompasses various components such as cardiovascular fitness, muscular strength and endurance, flexibility, and body composition. Maintaining good physical health is essential for countering early aging and promoting general well-being.

Role of Physical Health in Countering Early Aging

Prevents Chronic Diseases

Engaging in regular physical activity reduces the risk of chronic diseases like heart disease, type 2 diabetes, and certain types of cancer, which can contribute to premature aging.

Improves Cardiovascular Health

Regular exercise promotes a healthy heart by improving blood circulation, reducing blood pressure, and strengthening the cardiovascular system. This helps in preventing heart diseases that can speed up aging.

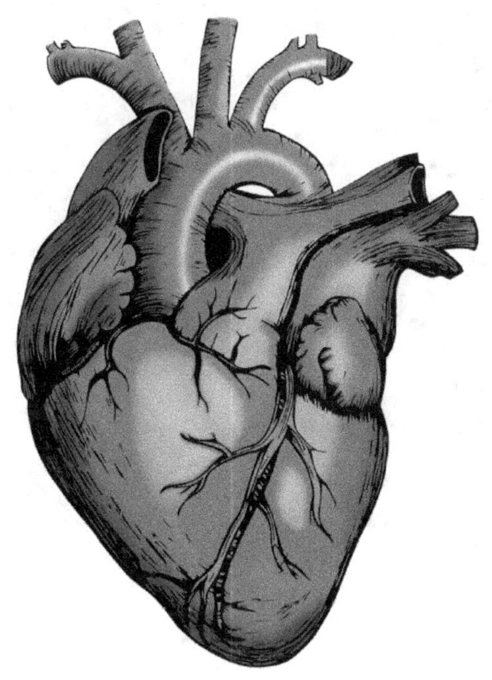

Boosts Immunity

Regular physical activity strengthens the immune system, making the body more resistant to illnesses and infections. This helps in reducing the impact of age-related decline in immunity.

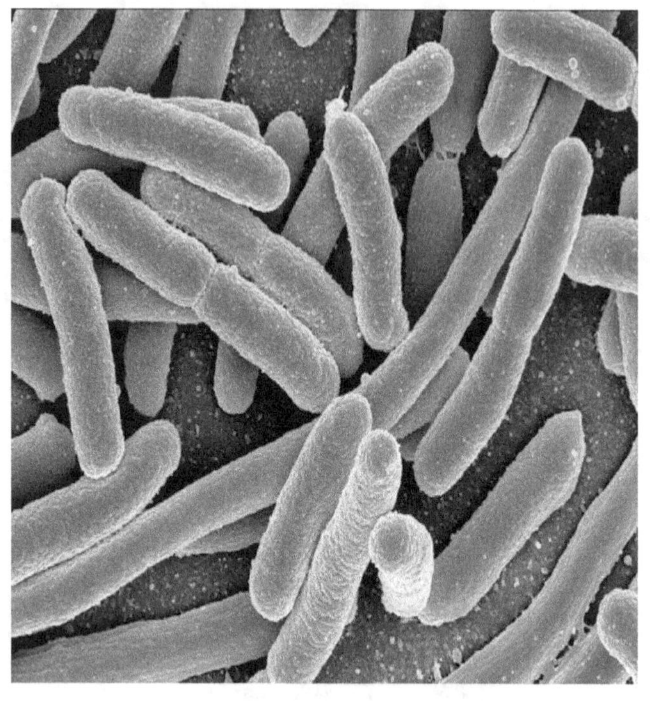

Maintains Cognitive Function

Physical exercise is associated with improved cognitive function and a reduced risk of cognitive decline. It helps in maintaining memory, mental acuity, and overall brain health, thus countering age-related cognitive decline.

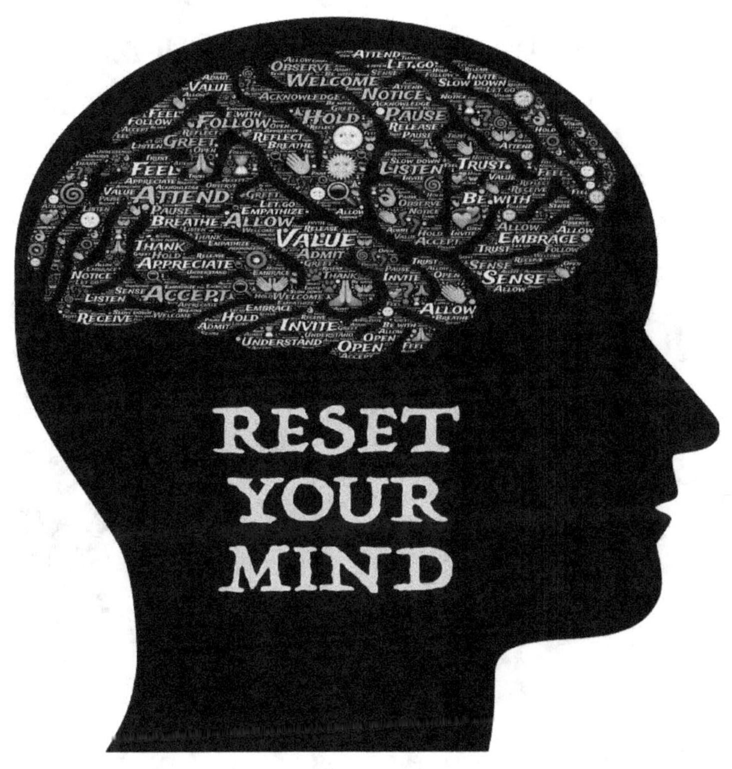

Preserves Muscle Mass and Bone Density

Regular strength training exercises can counteract age-related muscle loss (sarcopenia) and maintain bone density. This helps in preventing frailty, maintaining mobility, and reducing the risk of fractures.

Importance of Physical Health in Promoting General Well-being

Mental Health

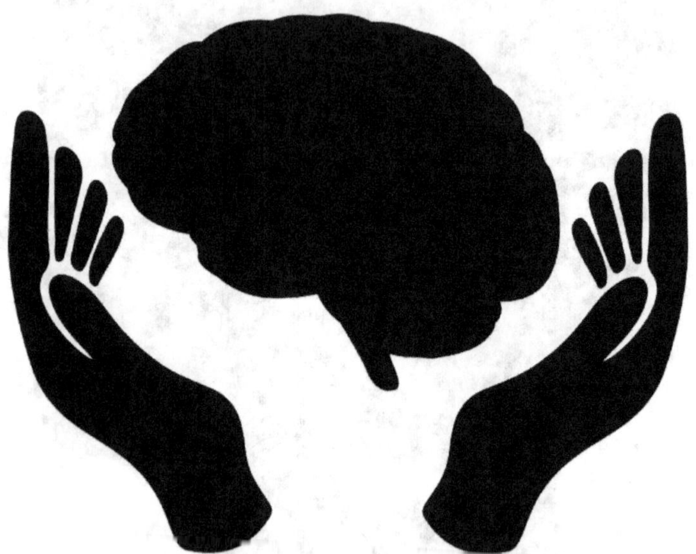

Regular exercise releases endorphins, which are natural mood boosters and help combat stress, anxiety, and depression. It promotes better sleep, reduces symptoms of mental health disorders, and enhances overall psychological well-being.

Practice stress operation ways, similar as awareness, deep breathing exercises, or contemplation.

Cultivate a positive mindset through gratefulness practices and positive tone- talk. Seek support from musketeers, family, or professionals in times of stress or emotional challenges.

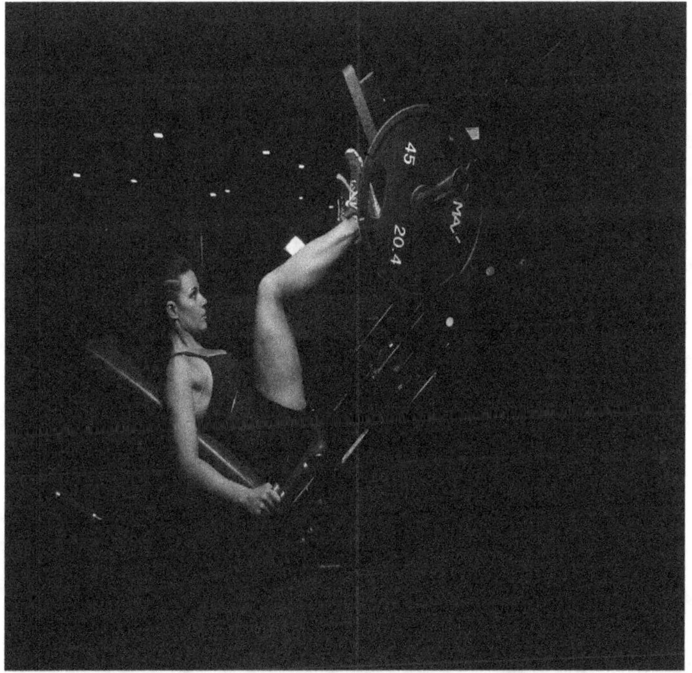

Physical activity increases energy levels, improves stamina, and enhances overall vitality. It helps in daily tasks, increases productivity, and enhances quality of life.

Engaging in regular physical activity helps in maintaining a healthy weight by burning calories and increasing metabolism. It reduces the risk of obesity and related conditions, improving overall well-being. Exercising regularly or engaging in regular physical exertion can benefit your skin and body by perfecting blood gyration, reducing stress, and boosting collagen product. Include a mix of cardiovascular exercises, strength training, and stretching in your routine.

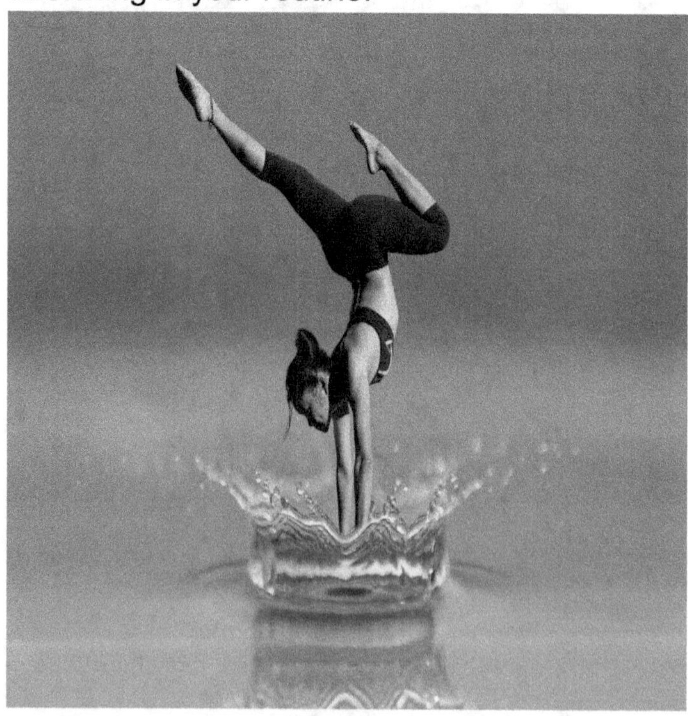

Manage Stress habitual stress can have mischievous goods on your skin and overall health. Practice stress operation ways like contemplation, deep breathing exercises, yoga, or hobbies that help you relax and relax.

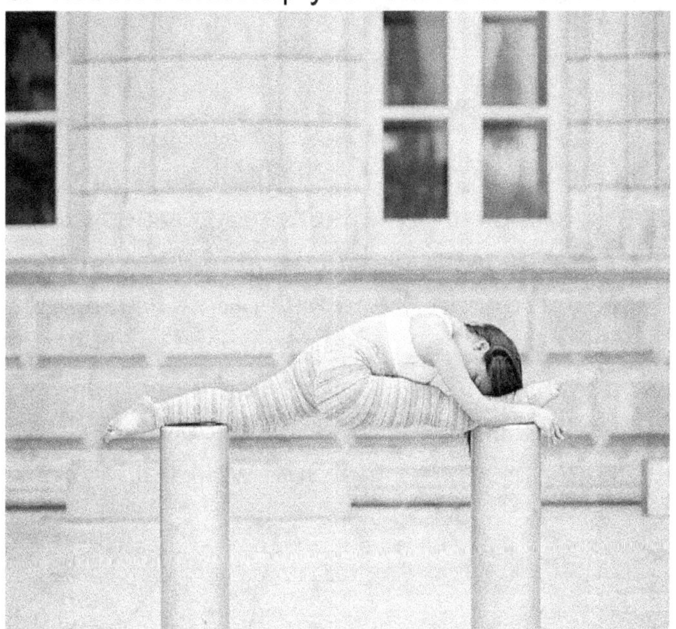

Quality of Life

Physical health directly impacts an individual's ability to perform daily activities and maintain an independent lifestyle. It enhances physical mobility, flexibility, and agility, thus improving overall quality of life. Stay active mentally keep your mind engaged by challenging yourself

intellectually. Engage in exertion like reading,
mystifications, learning new chops, or
participating in social relations to promote
cognitive health and maintain an immature
mindset.

Social Interaction

Participating in physical activities, such as
team sports or group exercises, provides
opportunities for social interaction, fostering a
sense of community and well-being. Maintain
Positive connections and compass yourself
with positive and supportive connections.
Good social connections can reduce stress
situations, promote emotional well- being and

contribute to overall life.

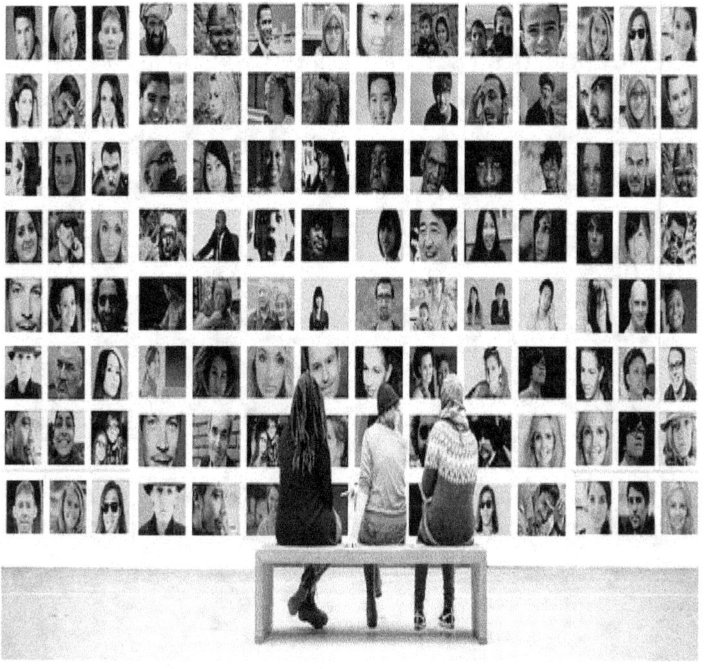

Nurture connections with family and
musketeers by spending quality time together,
engaging in meaningful exchanges, or
planning conditioning together. Join
community groups or associations that align
with your interests and values. Volunteer or
engage in acts of kindness to contribute to your
community and connect with suchlike- inclined
individualities. share in social gatherings or
events to expand your social network and
foster new connections.

Address any health enterprises beforehand on, perfecting the overall quality of your life as you age. Flash back, everyone's trip and experience with aging is unique. Embrace your individuality and make choices that align with what feels swish for your mind, body, and spirit.

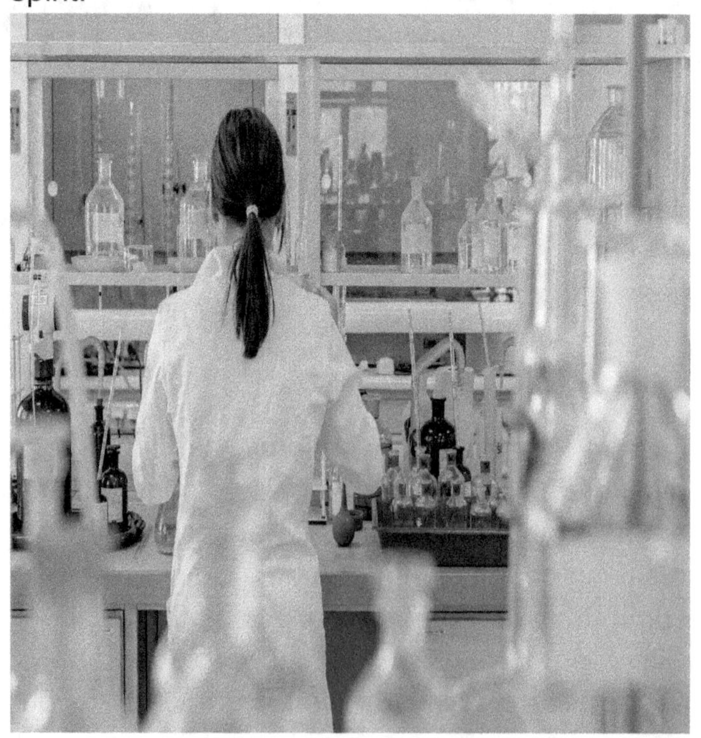

Maintain a Healthy Diet

A balanced diet rich in antioxidants, vitamins,
and minerals can help cover your skin and
body from aging. Include cornucopia of fruits,
vegetables, whole grains, spare proteins, and
healthy fats in your refections. Stay bedraggled
Keeping your body well- doused is vital for
maintaining healthy skin. Drink cornucopia of
water throughout the day to keep your skin
moisturized and to flush out venoms.
Engage in regular physical exercise, including
cardiovascular conditioning, strength training,
and inflexibility exercises. Get enough sleep to
promote physical and internal revivification.
Stay doused by drinking an acceptable
quantum of water throughout the day.
Schedule regular check- ups and preventative
wireworks to cover your physical health.

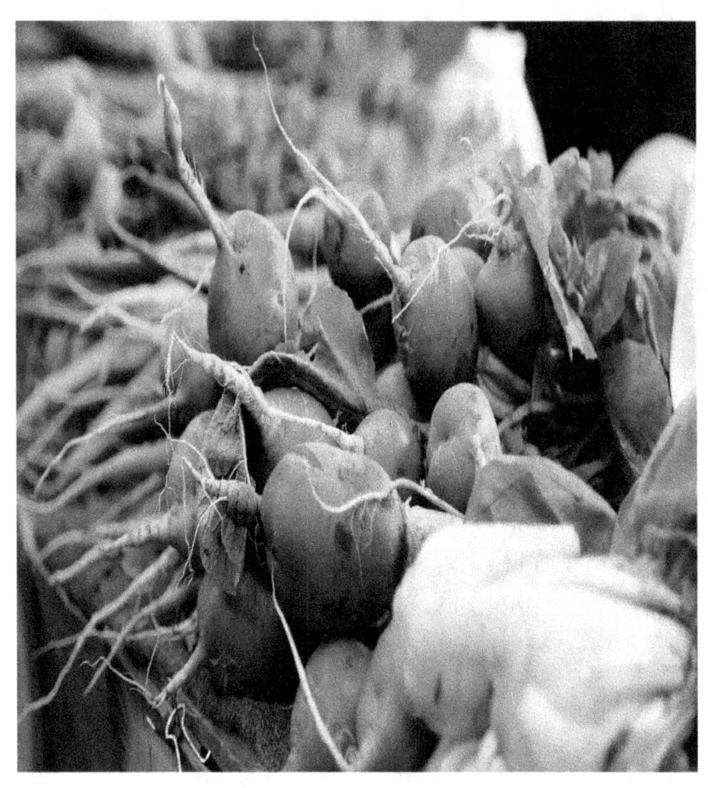

CHAPTER SIX

Cutting-Edge Anti-Aging Interventions

Telomere Lengthening

Telomeres are protective caps at the end of chromosomes that shorten with age. Telomere lengthening therapies, such as telomerase activation, aim to maintain or lengthen telomeres, potentially slowing down cellular aging.

Senolytics

Senescence is a state where cells are no longer functioning optimally and can contribute to aging. Senolytics are drugs or compounds that selectively target and eliminate senescent cells, promoting tissue rejuvenation.

Stem Cell Therapy

Stem cells have the potential to regenerate and repair damaged tissues. Stem cell therapies involve injecting stem cells into specific areas of the body to regenerate cells and tissues, potentially reversing some signs of aging.

Hormone Replacement Therapy

Hormones like testosterone and estrogen naturally decline with age. Hormone replacement therapy can help restore hormone levels to more youthful levels and alleviate symptoms associated with aging.

CHAPTER SEVEN

Natural Remedies to Slow Down Aging

Healthy Diet

Eating a balanced diet rich in antioxidants, vitamins, minerals, and omega-3 fatty acids helps protect against cellular damage and oxidative stress. Include plenty of fruits, vegetables, whole grains, lean proteins, and healthy fats in your diet.

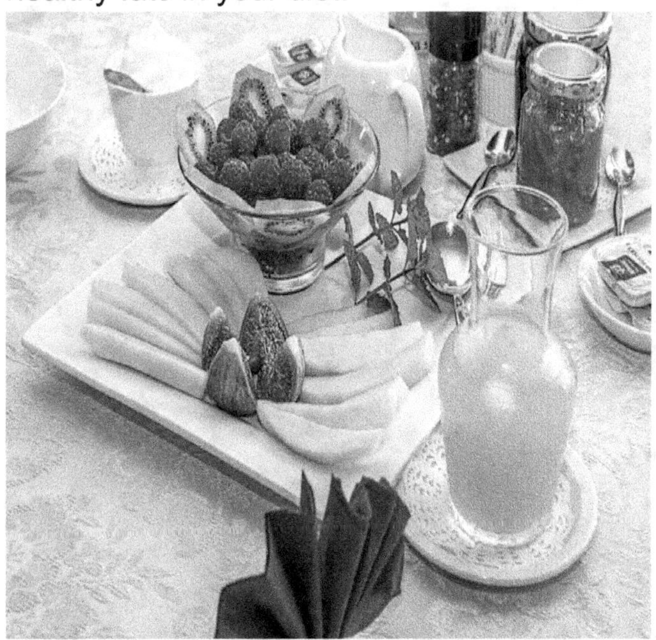

Exercise

Regular physical activity, including both cardiovascular and strength training exercises, can slow down the aging process. It improves circulation, strengthens muscles, improves flexibility, and enhances overall vitality.

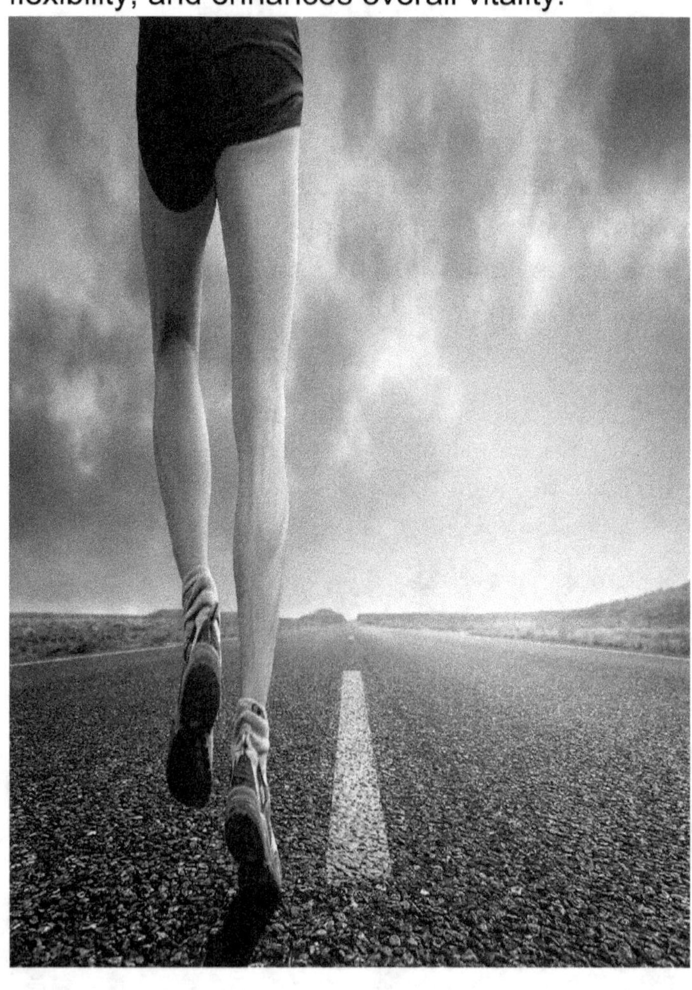

Chronic stress accelerates aging. Practice stress reduction techniques like meditation, deep breathing exercises, yoga, or engaging in hobbies, which promote relaxation and mental well-being.

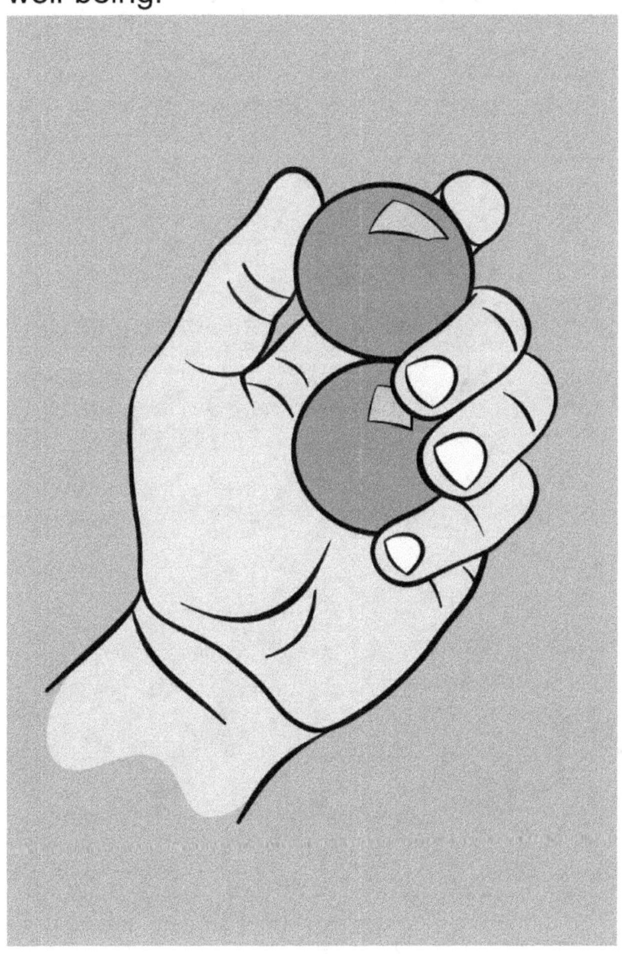

Adequate Sleep

Poor sleep quality and duration accelerate aging. Aim for 7-8 hours of quality sleep each night to promote cellular repair, cognitive function, and overall well-being wholesomeness and maintain immature skin

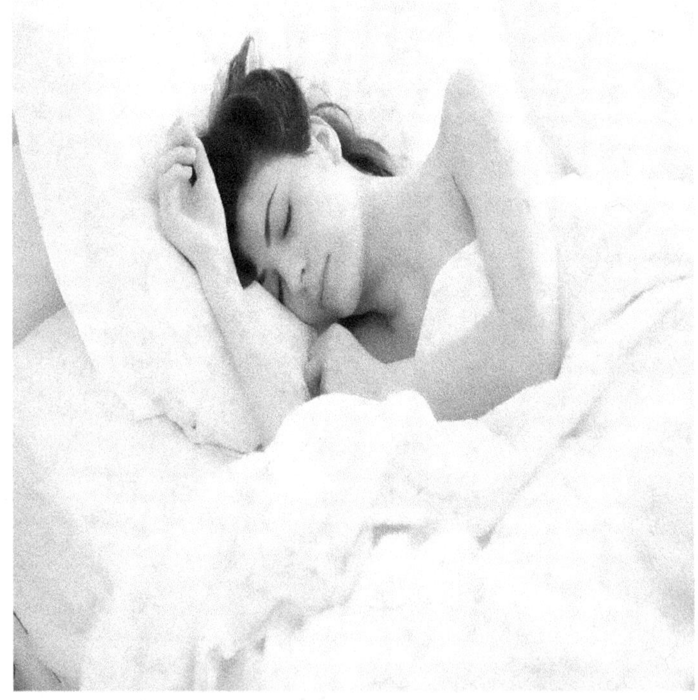

Sun Protection

Protect your skin from harmful UV radiation by wearing sunscreen, protective clothing, and sunglasses. Overexposure to the sun can accelerate skin aging and increase the risk of skin cancers. Protect your skin from Sun damage
Ultraviolet shafts from the sun can accelerate skin aging. Always wear sunscreen with a high SPF, indeed on cloudy days, and avoid prolonged sun exposure. Use protective vesture, wide- brimmed hats, and sunglasses to shield your skin from dangerous shafts.

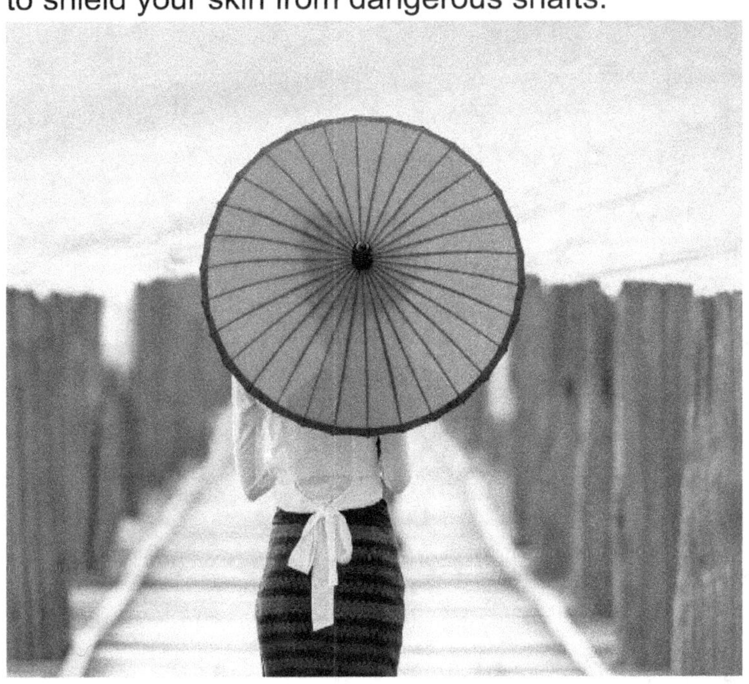

Furthermore, exercise a harmonious skincare routine cleanse your skin daily to remove dirt, oil painting oil, and makeup. Use a gentle cleanser suitable for your skin type. Follow up with a moisturizer to keep your skin doused. Consider incorporating anti- aging products, analogous as retinoids or serums, into your routine.

CHAPTER EIGHT

Practical Lifestyle Changes for Anti-Aging

Quit Smoking

Smoking accelerates aging and damages the skin. Quitting smoking not only improves overall health but also slows down premature aging. Avoid Smoking, smoking damages collagen and elastin fibers, causing premature wrinkles and growing skin. It's swish to avoid smoking.

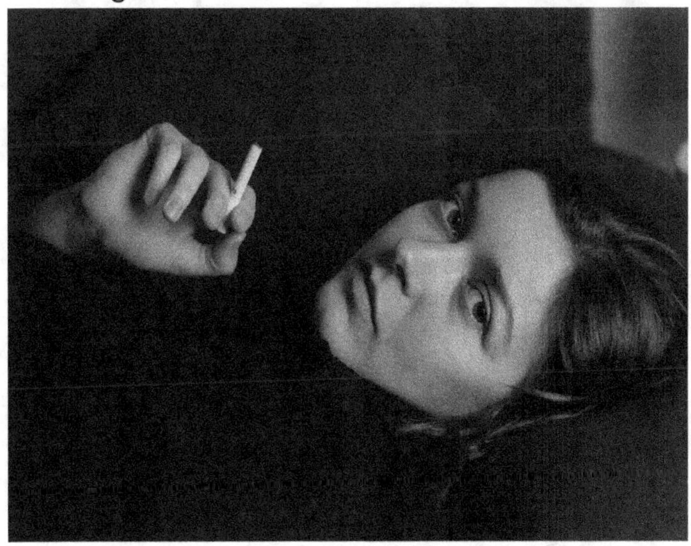

Limit Alcohol Consumption

Excessive alcohol consumption can lead to oxidative stress, inflammation, and liver damage. Limit alcohol intake or practice moderate drinking to slow down the aging process. Intake of devilish alcohol consumption can dehydrate your skin and lead to inflammation.

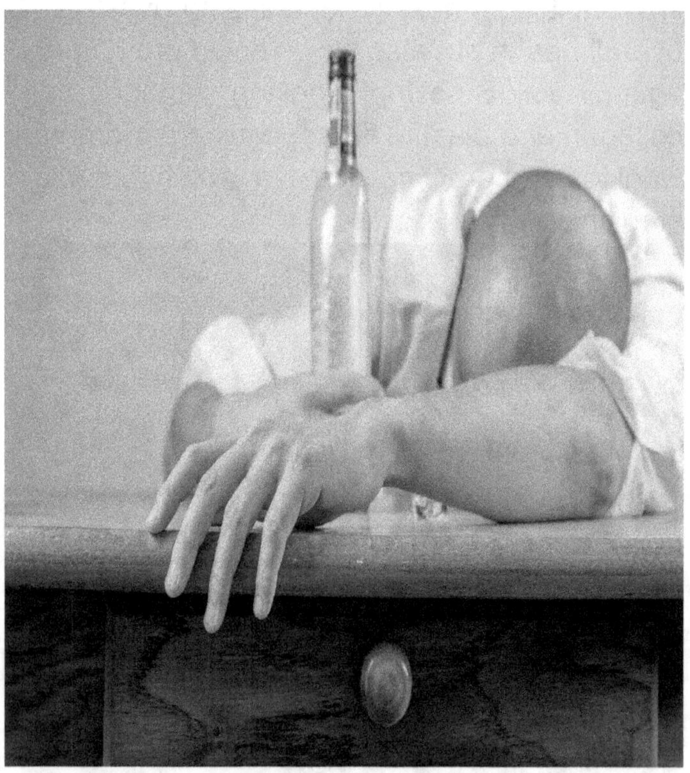

Maintain Hydration

Drink an adequate amount of water daily to promote healthy cellular function, skin hydration, and detoxification. Water is the fundamental basis in which all life are formed.

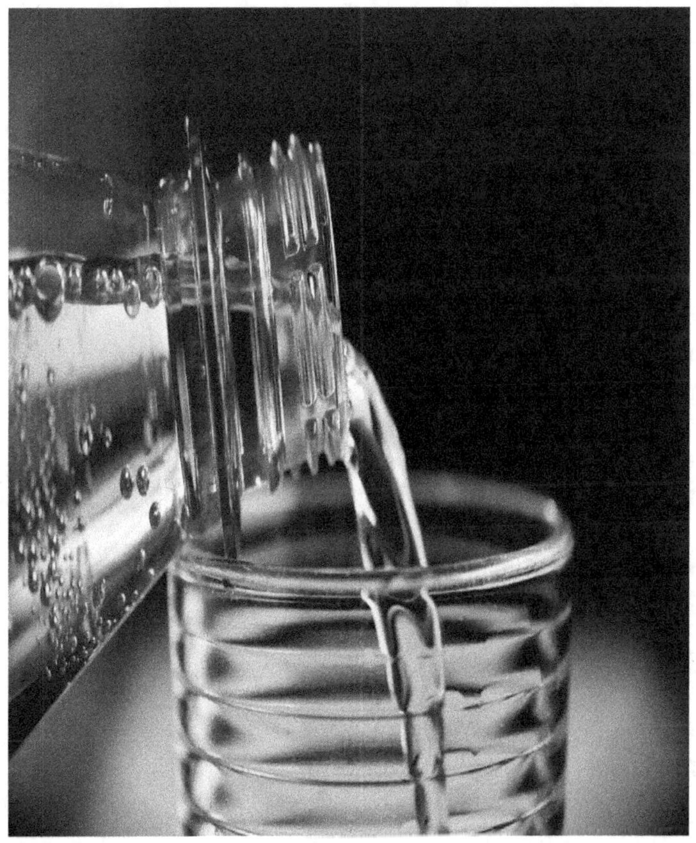

Mindful Skincare Routine

Follow a skincare routine that includes gentle cleansing, moisturizing, and protection from the sun. Use products containing antioxidants and ingredients that promote collagen production.

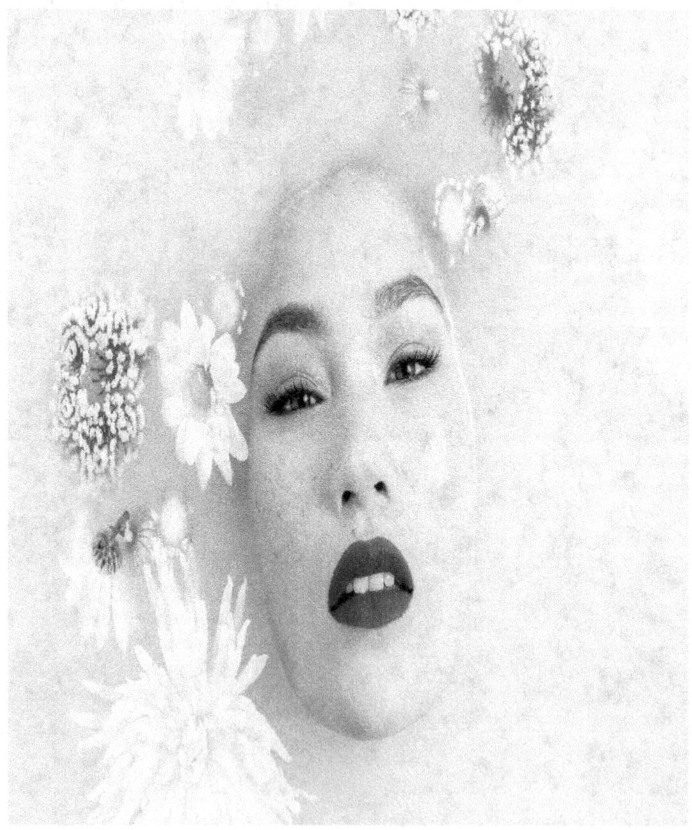

Social Engagement
Maintain a strong social network and engage in social activities regularly. Positive social connections have been associated with a slower aging process and improved overall well-being.

While cutting-edge anti-aging interventions offer promising advancements, natural remedies, and practical lifestyle changes remain fundamental in healthy aging. They can help slow down the aging process, promote overall well-being, and reduce the risk of age-related diseases. It's important to consult with healthcare professionals before considering any interventions or making significant lifestyle changes.

Flash- aging is a holistic approach that encompasses both external skincare and internal vitality. By espousing these comprehensive secrets, you can enhance your chances of growing gracefully and maintain a immature appearance.

CONCLUSION

In conclusion, the trip to fighting early aging and promoting general good is a multifaceted and dynamic path. Throughout this book, we've explored slice- edge anti-aging interventions, natural remedies, and practical life changes that can be enforced to decelerate down the aging process. By embracing the advancements in medical wisdom, we've uncovered remarkable interventions like telomere stretching, senolytics, stem cell remedy, and hormone relief remedy.

These slice- edge approaches hold immense eventuality for diving the underpinning mechanisms of aging and invigorating our cells, furnishing us with a renewed vigor and vitality. In parallel, we've dived into the significance of natural remedies that Mother Nature has bestowed upon us. From the power of a nutrient-rich diet and regular exercise to stress reduction ways, sleep hygiene, and sun protection, we've witnessed how these natural interventions nourish not only our bodies but also our minds, eventually enhancing our general good.

Still, let us not forget the significance of practical life changes in this narrative. Quitting smoking, limiting alcohol consumption, maintaining hydration, espousing aware skincare routines, and fostering social connections are all vital aspects of our trip towards fighting early aging and living a balanced, fulfilling life.

Therefore, the holistic approach to fighting early aging and promoting general good integrates the stylish of scientific improvements, natural remedies, and life variations. It's the community of these rudiments that empowers us to write our own narrative of graceful aging, embracing life's mannas with sprightliness and adaptability.

As we conclude this book, may it serve as a guiding light, inspiring you to take charge of your own health and good. Each small step, be it incorporating an antioxidant-rich mess, planning for many twinkles daily, or exploring slice- edge interventions with the guidance of healthcare professionals, has the implicit to produce a profound impact on how we progress and witness life.

Flash back, growing gracefully isn't solely about the number of times we accumulate, but the quality and sprightliness with which we live those times. So, let us embark on this transformative trip, armed with knowledge, determination, and an unvarying belief in our capability to nurture our bodies and minds, athwart beforehand growing, and embrace a life of optimal good.